The Ultimate Guide Intermittent Fasting For Women Over 50

Discover the Key To Delay Aging,
Boost Your Self-Esteem, And Feel
Fit By Eating Healthy With The
Intermittent Fasting Diet

Melisa Longer

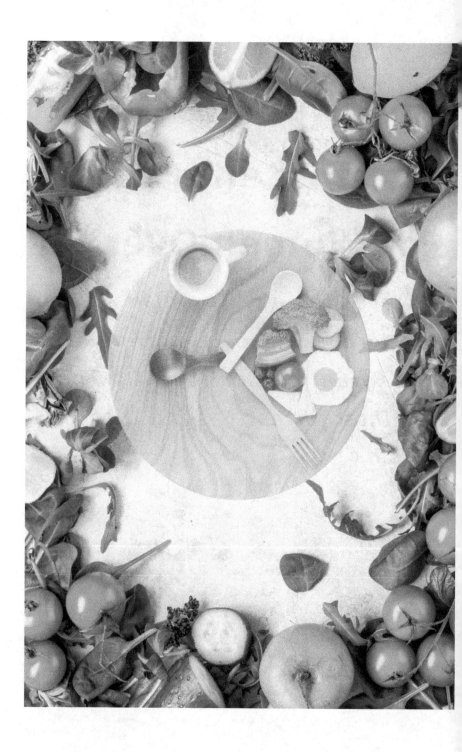

TABLE CONTENTS

—

Chapter One

How Intermittent Fasting Works?

Fasting essentially allows the body to use stored energy, such as consuming excess body fat.

It is vital to understand that this is normal and that humans have adapted to move without having to suffer adverse health effects. All energy from the food is contained in body fat. If you don't feed, the body can actually' use' its fat for energy.

Life is about equilibrium: the good and the bad.

By consuming more food, more energy than we can use is absorbed. Some of that energy needs to be retained for later use. Insulin is the principal hormone involved in the production of food energy.

This helps to store excess sugar when consuming insulin in two different ways. Sugars in long chains can bind glycogen, which is then stored in the liver. Nevertheless, storage space is small and once it is full, the liver begins converting excess glucose into fat. This cycle is called de novo lipogenesis (which means "re-creating fat").

Some of the newly created fat is retained in the liver but most of it is transferred to other body fat stores. Though this process is more complicated, the amount of fat produced has no limit. The body has two compatible feeding energy storage mechanisms. One is very easy to access, but it has a limited storage capacity (glycogen) and the other is the hardest to reach. Still, it does have an unlimited storage capacity (body fat.)

The cycle works in reverse when we don't eat (fasting). Insulin levels drop, allowing the body to start burning stored energy since it no longer receives food. Glucose in the blood drops, and the body must pump glucose from the tank to use it as fat.

Glycogen is energy's most open source. It breaks down into glucose molecules to provide energy to other cells. In this way, enough fuel can be supplied to the body for 24-36 hours. Instead, the body begins to break down to use fat as fuel.

So, the body can only be in two states: absorption (high insulin) and fasting (low insulin). Either we store the food energy, or we waste energy. It's one procedure or another. If there is a balance between eating and fasting, then there is no net weight gain.

When we begin to eat from the moment we get up and don't stop until we go to sleep, we spend most of the time in the state of absorption. We'll gain weight over time. We left no time to burn food energy to the body. To restore balance or lose weight, we simply need to increase the time we consume food energy. It is fasting. Fasting allows the body to use stored energy. After all, that is what it is about. You need to remember that nothing is wrong with this: that is how the body is designed. It's what dogs, cats, tigers, and bears do and we humans do.

When you eat regularly, as is often advised, the body uses the fuel from the food that comes in and does not consume the body fat, it will only store it. The body keeps it for when there is nothing to eat.

EFFECTS OF INTERMITTENT FASTING

Many investigations have studied the effects of intermittent fasting on the human body in some of its modalities. More research is needed but the results are very promising: intermittent fasting causes blood insulin levels to drop, particularly after 16 hours of fasting, making it easier to burn fat and increase the growth hormone that builds muscles, strengthens the immune system, and regenerates joints. Short-term fasting induces autophagy in the brain, a mechanism by which neurons kill their harm.

Restricting the amount of food in worms and rats, which can live twice as much, has shown to prolong life. It seems that intermittent fasting works the same way but without a miserable life of constant hunger. Fasting activates sit-ins, proteins that control inflammation and aging, protects cells from oxidation and prevent cancer cells' proliferation.

Intermittent fasting tends to increase insulin sensitivity, reducing glucose levels, and thus could be used to avoid type 2 diabetes.

This diet has been proven effective in reducing inflammation and oxidative stress, two of the trigger factors of cardiovascular disease.

Intermittent fasting decreases LDL cholesterol, raises cholesterol from HDL, reduces blood pressure and triglycerides, avoiding worse problems. It has succeeded in stopping Alzheimer's disease in rats. Also, nine of ten participants improved in a recent trial with human patients, thanks to the fasting program.

How to do it

It may not be easier to test the effects of intermittent fasting personally, but keep in mind these indications:

- Most of the fasting time at night is the most comfortable way. For example, the day you start, you usually eat at noon, and you no longer eat during the day. Skip breakfast the next day and eat at noon for the first time.
- Drink water as if tomorrow wasn't there. You can also drink tea, coffee, and any liquid with no calories in general. No, it's impossible to add honey to the tea.
- Start with a day of weekly fasting. For instance, if you acclimatize well on Tuesday and Friday, you can do it on two non-consecutive days.
- It is recommended that the day you start fasting should be a day off from your workout program. The next day's trend, exercise just before the first meal.
- Avoid prolonged fasting exercise. Take a small portion of protein, a shake, or amino acid tablets

containing leucine if you exercise strength or intervals, so you stop burning muscle mass.

Chapter Two

Best Types of Intermittent Fasting for Women Over 50

There is no one-size-fits-all strategy when it comes to dieting. This refers also to extended fasting.

In general, women should approach fasting more relaxed than men.

This could include shorter fasting times, fewer days of fasting, and eating a limited number of calories on fasting days.

Here are some of the best forms of female intermittent fasting:

- Crescendo method: fast from 12 to 16 hours for two or three days a week. Fasting days should be non-consecutive and evenly distributed throughout the week (e.g., Monday, Wednesday, and Friday).

- Eat (also called 24-hour protocol): a total fast of 24 hours once or twice a week (maximum twice a week for women). Start with fasts for 14 to 16 hours and gradually increase.
- Diet 5: 2 (also called "Quick Diet"): limit calories to 25% of the usual consumption (about 500 calories) for two days a week and eat "normally" for the other five days. Allow one day between fasting days.
- Modified fasting on alternate days: fasting on alternate days, but eating "normally" on days without fasting. It is allowed to consume 20 to 25% of the normal calorie intake (about 500 calories) on a fasting day.
- The 16/8 method (also called the "Lean gains method"): fast for 16 hours a day and eat all calories in an eight-hour window. Women are advised to start with a 14-hour fast and finally up to 16 hours.

Whatever your choice, during non-fasting periods, it is still essential to eat well. During the eating window, if you consume many unhealthy, high-calorie foods, you may not experience the same weight loss and health benefits.

The best approach is the one you can tolerate and sustain in the long run, which does not have adverse health consequences.

For women, there are many ways of doing intermittent fasting. The 5: 2 diet, modified alternative day fasting, and the growth method are some of the best techniques.

Chapter Three

Benefits of Intermittent Fasting Over 50
HEART HEALTH

Heart disease is the number one cause of death in the world. In turn, high blood pressure, high LDL cholesterol, and elevated triglyceride concentrations are some of the biggest risk factors for developing that condition.

A research of 16 overweight men and women found an elevated rate that reduced blood pressure by 6 percent in just eight weeks after following a fasting program.

.

Intermittent fasting in the same study decreased LDL cholesterol by 25% and triglycerides by 32%.

Nevertheless, the association between intermittent fasting and increased LDL cholesterol levels and triglycerides is not reliably clear.

Higher-quality studies with stronger methods are needed before researchers can fully understand the effects of intermittent fasting on heart health.

DIABETES

Intermittent fasting can also help manage and effectively reduce the risk of diabetes.

Some of the risk factors for diabetes appear to be reduced by intermittent fasting compared with extended caloric restriction.

This is done primarily by raising insulin levels and increasing insulin resistance.

In a randomized controlled study of more than 100 overweight or obese women, six months of intermittent fasting resulted in a 29% reduction in insulin levels and a 19% reduction in insulin resistance. There was no change in the blood sugar levels.

Besides, it has been shown those 8 to 12 weeks of intermittent fasting decreases insulin levels by 20 to 31 percent and blood sugar levels by 3 to 6 percent in people with prediabetes, a disorder in which blood sugar levels are normal, but elevated just enough to diagnose diabetes. Nevertheless, intermittent fasting may not be as beneficial for women in terms of blood sugar as it is for men.

A small study showed that blood sugar regulation decreased for women after 22 days of fasting in alternating days, while men had no adverse effect on blood sugar. Because of this side effect, decreasing insulin and insulin resistance will probably reduce the risk of diabetes, especially in patients with pre-diabetes.

WEIGHT LOSS

Intermittent fasting can be an easy and effective way to lose weight if done correctly, as regular short-term fasting can help you consume fewer calories and lose pounds.

Several studies suggest that intermittent fasting is as effective for short-term weight loss as conventional calorie-restricted diets.

A study of overweight adult research in 2018 showed that intermittent fasting resulted in an average weight loss of 6.8 kg (4 pounds approximately) over a 3 to 12-month period.

Another study found that intermittent fasting over 3 to 24 weeks in overweight or obese adults decreased body weight by 3 to 8 percent. The study also showed that participants decreased their waist diameter by 3–7 percent during the same period.

It should be recalled that the long-term effects of intermittent fasting on weight loss for women have not yet been shown.

In the short term, intermittent fasting appears to help you lose weight. However, how much you lose depends on how many calories you eat during times without fasting, and how long you stick to the lifestyle.

Chapter Four

The Seven Advantage of the Intermittent Fasting
ADVANTAGE ONE: YOU CAN ENJOY THE LITTLE PLEASURES
OF LIFE

Many diets recommend making the ice cream or dessert a definite cross. That's certainly good advice to lose weight. But putting it into practice is not easy. It goes on to abstain for six months or a year, but what about your remaining days? And then, why do you want to? Think a little over it. What could be more fun than sharing the assembled piece at your best friend's wedding and toasting with a glass of champagne? Want to abandon those pleasures forever? Instead of a birthday cake, choose a birthday salad? Existence loses its flavor a little bit, isn't it? There's a long time to live.

Fasting after occasional sprains helps restore balance. That is the essence of the cycle of life. Abundance carries on from drought. Starvation causes overflowing. It was always this way. Since time immemorial, feasts have always been celebrated with birthdays, weddings, parties, and other special occasions.

Nevertheless, such feasts must be accompanied by fasts. You can afford deviations by not eating as soon as you compensate them. Fasting is above all about equilibrium.

ADVANTAGE TWO: IT'S POWERFUL

Many people with type 2 diabetes are considered overweight and have marked insulin resistance. Sometimes even a strict ketogenic diet (very few carbohydrates, not too much protein, and lots of fat) is not sufficiently powerful to cope with the condition. Fasting is the easiest and most effective way of reducing insulin and improving insulin resistance in those situations. Fasting is powerful to conquer the stages during weight loss and raising the need for insulin.

The number of fasts that can be performed is not limited, and this is the main therapeutic benefit. The longest reported fast has lasted 382 days, with no detrimental effect on the patient. If it often happens that the fast doesn't yield the expected results, it's enough to increase the frequency or length until the target is achieved. By the way, diets—low in fat, low in carbohydrates (low carb,) or paleo—work for some people but not others. If you don't get any diet results, you'll have little leeway to make it more effective. On the other hand, with fasting, you just need to lengthen the time! The faster you go, the more likely you will lose weight, but it will always happen.

ADVANTAGE THREE: IT'S FLEXIBLE

Many diets recommend starting to eat in the morning, and then splitting meals by consuming the rest of the day every two-and-a-half hours. For some people, that type of diet works well. Nevertheless, finding and preparing something to eat six, seven, or eight times a day is extremely difficult. However, it is possible to go for 16 hours or 16 days at any time. There is no set deadline. You can fast one day a week, 5 days the next week, then 2 days the next. Fasting adapts to your responsibilities and enables several durations to be combined without being locked into a system.

If you live in the United States, the Netherlands, the United Arab Emirates, the polar Arctic desert, or Saudi Arabia's sandy desert, you can fast everywhere. Fasting makes your life simpler once again because you just have nothing to do. Where other proposals add complexity, it brings simplicity. If you don't feel well at some point in the fast, simply stop fasting. The malaise is going to go away.

ADVANTAGE FOUR: IT IS COMPATIBLE WITH ALL DIETS

The compatibility of fasting with all diets is its big asset. It does not impose any particular practice but, on the contrary, it consists of doing nothing.

- Are you not eating meat? This isn't stopping you from fasting.

- Are you not eating wheat? This isn't stopping you from fasting.

- Do you have an allergy to the dried fruit? This isn't stopping you from fasting.

- Short-term? This isn't stopping you from fasting.

- Are you running short? This isn't stopping you from fasting.

- Are you always on the go? This isn't stopping you from fasting.

- You're not sure how to cook? This isn't stopping you from fasting.

- Are you eighty-five years old? This doesn't deter you from fasting.

- Do you have difficulty chewing? This isn't stopping you from fasting.

ADVANTAGE FIVE: IT'S SIMPLE

Lack of consensus about what constitutes a healthy diet also creates patient uncertainty. Is there a low-fat diet they should be on? Down with carbohydrates? Under-calorie? Down with sugar? Low on the glycaemic index? A radically different fasting approach makes it easier to understand. Two sentences suffice to describe it. Nothing to sleep. Drink water, tea, bone broth, or coffee.

That's all; diets can fail because of ineffectiveness, but also because they're not properly followed up. The most obvious advantage of fasting is its simplicity, which is the main reason for its effectiveness. The easier the better when it comes to the dietetic laws.

ADVANTAGE SIX: IT'S FREE

Of course, in an ideal world, everyone would eat organic vegetables and organic beef that had grazed near them instead of white bread or highly processed food. The fact remains that sometimes these organic foods will cost up to 10 times more than that of industrial food.

The government subsidizes cereals, making them far more competitive than other foods. For this reason, a kilo of cherries can cost 8$ or 9$, while a baguette is worth about 1$ and even less a packet of pasta. Feeding a family of pasta and white bread over a tight budget is much simpler.

No matter how efficient a scheme is when its costs are prohibitive. The price makes it unaffordable for those who can afford it. This should not allow them to have type 2 diabetes and its limitations.

Fasting is free. In reality, it doesn't just cost zero, it saves you money as you don't have to buy food at all! No expensive goods. No overpriced food supplement. No meal substitute or medicine. It's gratis.

ADVANTAGE SEVEN: IT'S PRACTICAL

Eating uncooked raw foods on your own is good for your health. Most people, however, have neither the time nor the inclination to make food every day. Time is the center of work, education, family, children, extracurricular activities, and personal activities. Cooking takes time: shopping, preparing the meal, without forgetting the time to cook and the time to clean it all. It takes time for everything,

---

and time is a scarce commodity that is usually sorely lacking.

Even if it is with the best intention in the world, advising everyone to cook isn't the best strategy if you really want to get results. Fasting, by contrast, is the exact opposite: more shopping, more preparation ingredients, cooking, and cleaning. It's a way of simplifying your life. Fasting itself is convenient. Nothing to do. Many schemes give directions. Fasting needs nothing. Keeping it easier is hard!

Chapter Five

Follow a Fast Schedule
LITTLE BY LITTLE FOLLOW THE INTERMITTENT FASTING DIET

If you're not used to fasting, your appetite, thirst, and body system may be influenced by this diet. You will follow it slowly if you extend the hours of fasting between meals or if you start avoiding food entirely on one day of the week. This will help your body to detoxify and decrease the painful symptoms (such as nausea, low blood pressure, exhaustion, or irritability) that you feel.

At the start of this diet, you can also eat light snacks during fasting times. A 100-calorie protein and a fat snack (such as nuts, cheese, etc.) won't affect how well you start and keep fasting. So, you could eat some very light snacks.

As part of this process, you will need to gradually modify your diet to reduce your consumption of processed foods such as processed meats, milk, or soda.

EAT YOUR LAST MEAL BEFORE YOU MAKE A FAST

Avoid the temptation of eating junk food, sugar, and processed foods in your last meal before fasting. Eat fresh fruits and vegetables, and plenty of protein, to maintain high levels of energy. For starters, your last meal could be a cooked chicken breast, a piece of garlic bread, and a salad made with roman lettuce, tomato, onion slices, and vinaigrette.

At the beginning of this method, some people eat compulsively but this will allow them to devote more time to food processing and less time to the "process of adaptation to fasting" of the food withdrawal period.

Eat a full meal until you start fasting. When you fill up before fasting, eating only sugar-rich foods and carbohydrates, you'll quickly feel hungry again. If you have a meal in your schedule, eat plenty of protein and fat. You might find it hard to maintain a very low intake of carbohydrates and fat, as you will always feel unhappy and hungry during the fast.

FAST DURING THE HOURS YOU SLEEP

If you do a long fast, it will be useful not to think about the stomach's sounds. Every night you should sleep for at least 8 hours; fast for at least a couple of hours while awake or sleeping. That way, you won't feel deprived of food when you wake up because you will consume a hearty meal soon.

Upon fasting, the first meal or main course you eat will be your fasting reward. You'll feel hungry, so you should eat a full meal.

Keep Your Body Well Hydrated

You're going to fast most hours of the day if you adopt an intermittent fasting diet, but that doesn't mean you can stop drinking water. Besides, it will be important to stay hydrated during fasting to ensure your body's proper functioning. Drink calorie-free water, herbal teas, and other beverages.

This will also keep you from feeling hunger pain, as the liquids will fill the abdomen area.

Fasting and the Hormones

Fasting is known to be healthy, especially therapeutic fasting, intermittent fasting, and long-term fasting. Various ailments are alleviated; some illnesses are cured.

But what influence does a fasting period have on the hormonal balance? What happens to our hormones while we are fasting? Will fasting lead to aging faster because some nutrients may be missing?

Usually, one does not want to admit that aging is a part of our lives, but it affects every individual, with some being caught up with the aging process a little earlier, others later. At least that's the thesis.

It has become known that the reduction in the production of certain hormones begins around the age of 40 and is a major cause of aging. Regular fasting can have significant positive effects and largely reduce the signs of aging.

But what are the hormones on which, for example, 16/8 interval fasting has such a beneficial influence? Can you make general use of this knowledge? Is it possible to have a way of life where the negative influences of aging can be stopped?

OUR HORMONES INFLUENCE ALL PROCESSES IN THE BODY

Hormones determine our rhythm of life, whether it is growth, puberty, aging, inner balance, and even our health. In all areas of our life, hormones are involved in essential processes in the organism.

The proportion of the hormone DHEA produced in the adrenal glands begins to decline at the age of 25.

Pronounced dehydroepiandrosterone, or DHEA for short, slows down the metabolism, reduces fat, and lowers blood pressure.

The two opponents are serotonin and adrenaline, which keep each other in check, are mostly known. With the stress hormone cortisol, which wants to convert everything into energy and makes sense in demanding situations, the DHEA slows down the increased energy burn and ensures a balanced energy balance.

You can visualize it like yin and yang, an image that stands for balance. If the production of DHEA drops, cortisone will likely gain the upper hand, which negatively affects the aging process.

But the sex hormones estrogen, progestin, and testosterone also decrease from around the age of 40. They are part of the tissue-maintaining and rejuvenating hormones. Other important hormones are serotonin and melatonin, the production of which also declines with age.

A list of important hormones that are involved in the aging process - or rather, it's slowing down:

- Serotonin (happiness hormone)
- Melatonin (sleep hormone)
- Estrogen (female cycle)
- Progestin (for water retention, female hormone)
- Testosterone (male sex hormone)
- Growth hormone STH (for body fat and muscle regulation)
- DHEA (slows down the metabolism)

On the other hand, adrenaline, noradrenaline, cortisol, and insulin (stress hormones) are unfavorable.

Chapter Six

What Happenes to The Hormones During Fasting

It is known that fasting has a positive effect on diseases such as rheumatism, arthritis, or osteoarthritis. This is related to an increase in the hormone cortisone administered in an artificial form in these diseases to curb the inflammation in the joints.

It is a reaction of the organism to the switch to the ketone metabolism, which initially means stress for the body. However, this diminishes as the fast continues and the cortisol level drops.

As the level of cortisol falls, so does the production of rejuvenating hormones such as DHEA and the growth hormone STH. The latter is even responsible for the fact that instead of muscle mass, fat tissue is broken down, which is very important in getting older. Because even from a distance, based on a person's silhouette, you can tell whether it is a young or older person.

Older people usually gain weight and build up fat deposits on the stomach, while at the same time losing muscle mass. This can lead to serious postural disorders and at some point, prevents you from getting up from the chair by yourself.

The sleep/happiness hormones melatonin and serotonin also boost their production to an appropriate extent during fasting. Especially in spring, the well-known springtime tiredness is quickly overcome with an internal spring cleaning through a fasting cure.

The serotonin level rises and the hormone melatonin ensures a particularly good sleep at night, which is also the cornerstone of a slowed down aging process.

THE POSITIVE EFFECTS OF FASTING ON OUR BODY AND THE HORMONE BALANCE AT A GLANCE

It is amazing how positively our body reacts to fasting in many different ways and how fasting hormones control us:

- Weight loss and the state of ketosis lower blood sugar levels and regulate insulin production.
- Lowering cholesterol and thus lowering the inflammatory parameters and strengthening the cardiovascular system.
- Strengthening the entire immune system with improved digestion and the associated defense against tumors and infections.
- Increasing in rejuvenating hormones like DHEA or STH and decreasing the stress hormones adrenaline and cortisol.
- Increasing the well-being and a good mood thanks to the happiness hormone serotonin.

- Improvement of sleep quality through a balanced melatonin balance, resulting in increased stress resilience in everyday life.
- Improvement and balance of the necessary sex hormones, such as estrogens and testosterone also have a rejuvenating effect on men's and women's bodies and minds.

FASTING HORMONES - THE BOTTOM LINE

Regular fasting cures positively influence the body, regardless of your age or health situation.

Therapeutic fasting cures or intermittent fasting have a rejuvenating effect. But not only that, the hormonal balance is a very complex system, which can be unbalanced by stress or poor nutrition.

An annual fast is the best option here. Possible complaints and illnesses can certainly be associated with a disturbed hormonal balance, which can be brought back into balance by a regular fasting period.

It is not for nothing that many people see their younger, firmer skin, a special glow of the eyes, and shiny hair after the fast.

It is not a free ticket to eternal life. Still, fasting offers a completely natural opportunity to live happily and healthily with aging and at the same time with a balanced hormone balance, no matter what phase of life you are in.

Chapter Seven

Lose Weight through an Intermittent Fasting Diet

Intermittent weight loss from fasting is a technique that has become popular over the past few years. It's a method of eating where you switch from feeding to fasting. You get to schedule your times of fasting and non-fasting, in which you drink only water. Although it is unnecessary to do intermittent fasting every other day to lose weight, it is advised for those who want to lose weight, at least twice a week.

With an intermittent fasting diet, you are allowed to eat anything you wish in the periods when you are not fasting. You'll stick to healthy foods if you're looking to lose weight and avoid those that will defeat the whole process purpose. During this time, it is recommended consuming carbohydrates as they help with fat metabolism.

Drinking water is highly encouraged when you are fasting, as staying hydrated helps you lose weight more quickly. After all, you can go without food for days, but not without water.

Over the years, fasting has helped many people lose weight, and keep it off. There are a lot of reasons why it's one of the easiest ways to get into shape. If you cut your calories by continuing through scheduled fasting times, the body is forced to provide nutrition from its reserves, usually fat. Because weight loss means eating less than you're consuming, fasting lets you focus more on exercise than on a diet.

With intermittent fasting, you get relative freedom with what you eat. This is different from the many fad diets where you're limited to certain types of food. Although freedom is provided, you should only take what's right for you, as mentioned earlier. Include plenty of fiber in your diet, as it means that your body is fully working. You have to establish and stick to some sort of plan for intermittent fasting to lose weight to work. A present intermittent fasting diet plan is hard to follow, as it might not work into your lifestyle. Instead, set your days of fasting and non-fasting.

To get the hang of intermittent fasting and how weight loss happens in the everyday lifestyle with its definition, here is a summary of how to do it and take advantage of it.

CHOOSE THE 24 HOURS IF TECHNIQUE OR 12-HOUR WINDOW

It is possible to agree on several forms of intermittent fasting cycles, some differ from 24 hours plus eating on Tuesday at 6 pm and then taking the next meal on Wednesday at 6 pm. This fast shouldn't be marketed as such for long as it impacts the metabolic rate and deteriorates health in turn. The best option is to choose a 12-hour period, where fasting takes place for half a day, and then consume any fat or carbohydrate food beneficial to the body.

What happens when one meal is taken is that the body uses it until the next 12 hours and the calorie stored as fat is consumed and employed by the body when digested. It results in weight loss, and after a while, the desire and hunger pangs will also vanish as the body becomes used to it.

KEEP THE DIET SIMPLE AND SHORT

Weight loss through intermittent fasting occurs only when it is regularly practiced. There should be a plan for consistency that is simple and easily followed daily. Set food groups at intervals of 12 hours, and just have those. A simple balance of the groups will decide the intake of food necessary for the well-being of the body, healthy metabolism, and ultimately weight burning out unexpectedly. Calcium, sugar, carbohydrates, and fats can be found in the community. The only thing to do is manage it properly.

REDUCES STRESS ON THE BODY NEEDING TO SNACK TIME AND AGAIN

Intermittent fasting molds the body's needs in a way where regular snacking needs naturally die down. What happens is when extra meal intake and fat were stored in the body, that particular time is simply cut off from the daily routine and weight loss begins to occur with it. The stress the body takes in the production, absorption and use of the food, and extra meal in the consumption is also decreased. Instead, the same amount of energy is used to absorb the stored calories and burn it down by reducing fat on the stomach other body parts.

BLOOD SUGAR LEVELS AND ROUTINES ARE ADJUSTED APPROPRIATELY

Intermittent fasting has several benefits and one of them is healthy blood sugar levels as the body's intake decreases. Studies show that fewer cravings occur and this type of diet also regulates blood pressure, stress, and heart disease. Not only would intensive workouts be avoided and drastic diet cuts would not occur, but eating just about everything you want and still weight reduction happens in a span of a few months. Also, more healthy food and nutrient intake develops as a habit over a period, something that is tough to make when IF is not followed.

Chapter Eight

The Importance of Exercise as Lifestyle

A physically active lifestyle is comparable to youth's fountain: it is one of the secrets to living longer, healthier, and happier.

Stress, along with general well-being, can be controlled through physical activity, and this is essential for achieving and maintaining a healthy body weight and reducing the risk of chronic diseases.

Among the benefits attributable to the practice of regular physical exercise, here are the main ones:

- It reduces stress.
- It improves self-esteem, self-control, and a sense of general well-being.
- It helps you keep fit.

- It helps to strengthen bones, muscles, and joints.
- It increase muscle strength and endurance.
- It allows to control the bodyweight.
- It reduces the risk of chronic diseases (vascular diseases, some cancers, type 2 diabetes mellitus).
- It improves the regulation of blood pressure in hypertensive and glycemic balance in diabetics.
- It reduces states of anxiety and depression.

Physical activity and nutrition are the two most important lifestyle variables for health. Staying active increases the amount of energy consumed, which is essential for weight control. As you age, your metabolism slows down, so you need to eat less and move more to keep your energy balance constant.

IMPLEMENTATION OF PHYSICAL ACTIVITY

Incorporating into the daily routine of a constant and moderate physical activity induces a series of physiological changes in the organism that go beyond burning calories, reducing fat, and maintaining muscle mass. In addition to promoting weight loss and improving the relationship between food and the body itself, physical activity induces a change in the body's composition and the functioning of metabolism and systems (circulatory, respiratory, etc.)

Daily physical exercise, for example, is a way to improve cardiovascular health because it acts on different fronts:

- It reduces blood pressure, favoring the control of hypertension.
- It increases the secretion of HDL cholesterol (good cholesterol), reducing the rate of blood cholesterol.
- It induces a decrease in triglyceride levels.
- It decreases the production of insulin, helping to control type 2 diabetes,

favoring the assimilation of nutrients, their arrival in the cells of the different tissues, and reducing the uptake and accumulation of fat.

PHYSICAL ACTIVITY

Control of cardiovascular risk factors (hypercholesterolemia, arterial hypertension, and type 2 diabetes).

- Increased lung capacity.
- Increase in muscle strength and mass.
- Increase in aerobic capacity.
- Reduction of fat mass.

It improves the person's psychological balance by inducing a state of personal satisfaction and the control of anxiety and stress.

Finally, it is worth highlighting the last benefit of physical activity. It improves the individual's relationship with food, reduces appetite, and favors the adoption of healthy eating habits.

We have to warn that in no way the IF approach can replace a direct health care provider, nor should it be used to determine a diagnosis, or to choose a procedure in particular cases.

Chapter Nine

What Are the Best Types of Exercises for You (Woman Over 50)?

It is time to set the table, but the exercises from 50 should be to get a healthy body. The following exercises work several muscles in your body, as well as the buttocks and hamstrings for women over 50, create stronger legs, thinner and with more force, to lift your rear part, the quadriceps also work, since they require that the knee to get resistance.

To perform the first of these exercises, stand in front of a bench or a firm chair and place your left foot firmly on top of the bench or chair. Press your left foot and push the body back until the left leg is straight; lower the body down until the right knee is flexed and repeat 10 to 15 times. Weight balanced evenly; don't lean too far forward or too far back.

The so-called bridge exercises are not only the perfect exercise for a perfectly rounded back, but they will also help women keep their back healthy and pain-free.

DEFINE ABS FOR WOMEN

To do this great exercise called a bridge, lie down on the floor with your face up, with your knees slightly bent and with your feet flat on the floor. Raise your hips so that your body shapes will take a curved line from the shoulders to the knees. Pause in the upper position for two or three seconds, then lower your body back to the initial position. Repeat this movement 10 to 15 times; then take a short rest of five minutes maximum and repeat the number of times before recommended.

ROUTINE ABDOMINALS FOR WOMEN

The addition of raising an arm while performing the previous exercise on the floor improves the posture and the strength of the base, which makes me feel better. It will seem more effort, but you will feel more secure.

Given the situation of reducing our belly, it is important to perform the exercises constantly and linearly; it is advisable to expand the abdominal table for women progressively. Every 10 or 15 days would be correct because each time we will have the most strengthened abdominal area.

STRENGTHEN BUTTOCKS

To perform the following exercise for women over 50 to create stronger, stronger legs and buttocks, start by adopting an iron position, but bend your elbows and lean on your forearms instead of on your hands.

EXERCISE TABLE FOR THE BUTTOCKS

Your body should create a straight line to the ankles from the shoulders. Tighten your buttocks and maintain your hip position while raising your right arm forward; move your shoulder blades down and back as you raise your arms. Keep the position for 5 to 10 seconds; relax the buttocks and repeat the exercise ten to fifteen times, alternating arms.

Yoga has so many physical and mental benefits. The postures are excellent to help reduce the appearance of cellulite. Make shoulder support or put your legs above the wall for 5 minutes every night before going to bed. This will be beneficial not only for the appearance of cellulite but also to collaborate greatly with leg circulation.

EXERCISES FOR WOMEN OVER 50 YEARS TO CREATE STRONGER, THINNER, AND STRONGER LEGS

To correctly perform the following exercise after 50, you have to take it more calmly. To create stronger, more firm legs and buttocks, lie on your back and gradually lift your hips and legs off the floor, bringing your legs above your head until your toes touch the ground behind you. Place your hands behind your back and extend your legs stretching them in the air, creating a straight line from your shoulders to your ankles. Keep your neck relaxed and your shoulder support hold, try to hold the position for at least one minute and then slowly reach the starting position, pause, rest, and then repeat the movement about ten more times, obviously with your respective breaks.

For a quick toning of the whole body, go through the movements described above and perform three sets of exercises about ten times or otherwise indicated by a medical condition; move as quickly as possible between the movements to the maximum calorie intake.

The next day, do other exercises. You can incorporate a few series of cardio intervals at the time of training your entire body; or you can do it separately over a longer period in these exercises for women over 50 years.

If you want to reinforce a specific part of your body, you should focus on exercises that train those particular muscles and incorporate them into your daily regimen. To continue to be effective, you should gradually increase the number of repetitions concerning how strong the muscle gets.

AN EXERCISE ROUTINE FOR WOMEN OVER 50

Multidirectional exercises help develop coordination and control while providing toning and hardening of the quadriceps, buttocks, hamstrings, and inner thighs.

EXERCISES AFTER 50 WILL HELP KEEP YOUR BACK HEALTHY AND PAIN-FREE

To perform the following exercise, stand with your feet together, both arms stretched over your head, palms facing forward. Take a wide step with your right foot towards the corner of the room at a 45-degree angle and diagonally, bending the right knee and reaching the lower part of your body in a forward motion on your right thigh. The back leg should be straight, with your heel lifted off the floor.

LEG AND BUTTOCK EXERCISES

If you can touch the ground, do it on both sides of your right foot, lightly with your fingers. Push with your right foot to return to the starting position. Repeat 15 times on one leg and 15 times for the other. An option to modify this exercise is not to go so low in the stride and aim to reach with your hands at the knee or the level of the shin instead.

LEG EXERCISES FOR WOMEN

As quick advice, stand again out of the position described above and focus on working out the abdominals with tight buttocks, squeezing your thighs together, and maintaining good posture.

In addition to getting thinner and stronger legs, the postures that we must adapt maintain a healthy and erect back. In addition to hardening our legs, our day to day will have a better quality of life. Now I remember what it cost to climb the stairs with a smile from ear to ear.

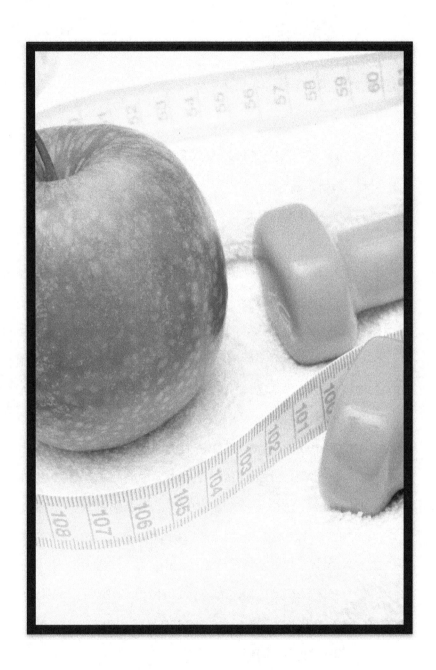

CHAPTER Ten

HEALTH BENEFITS WITH INTERMITTENT FASTING

FASTING AND CANCER

More and more scientists are trying to help cancer patients aim to change the oncological metabolic process to traditional treatments (chemotherapy, radiotherapy, surgery). In recent years, studies have been reported in which at the time of intermittent fasting in both animals and humans the modulating effects at the stage of metabolism were observed. Several volunteers underwent a study. The medical team discovered how glucose-insulin levels and, most importantly, the IGF-1 values (which is a potential oncological marker) and other cardiovascular risk indicators were greatly improved by fasting.

INTERMITTENT FAST CONFECTION

It is focused on having enough fasting hours from the last to the first intake of the next day, distributing amounts of glucose, insulin, inhibiting the mTOR's anabolic pathway, and activating the autophagic pathway of the AMPK. It has been noted that this starts to happen after 12 hours of fasting, although the ideal is to arrive between the last meal and the first intake of the next day until 14-16 hours of fasting.

The instructions to follow depend on each person's schedules and customs, but the intermittent fasting rule, in general, suggests that after getting up there must be 3-4 hours in which no food has been consumed, thereby increasing the glucose levels. Insulin and gluconeogenesis hormones (adrenaline, norepinephrine, glucagon, growth hormone, and cortisol) will be released; t4 to t3 conversion will be favored and free testosterone bioavailability will be improved in the early morning hours. This will encourage the triggering of the autophagic route at the start of the day and mobilize the accumulated fatty acids in the visceral fat adipocytes.

Upon getting up, the first intake would be 3-4 hours. Some people take the opportunity to do their first fasting training. They do it with low glucose and a lot of insulin sensitivity, which encourages a high-fat energy mobilization, with high lipolysis and induced thermogenesis because glucose is very small when training starts. One hour and a half or two hours before exercise are advised to make the first intake in other situations. To extend the activation of the AMPK route, this first intake should consist of protein and fat, particularly with medium-chain triglycerides found in coconut oil. In this way, the mitochondrial activity that works very efficiently from the medium-chain triglycerides will be very high.

Following the general guidance, carbohydrate intake should be done once the first practice is completed, thus breaking the AMPK route's function and activating the MTOR route linked to insulin receptor activation hyper expression of the body's proteins. Because of this super-compensation mechanism and improved insulin sensitivity in the previous 14-18 hours, the person can assimilate the carbohydrate much better and generate a beneficial impact through insulin, enabling him to refill better glycogen and activate the routes intended for tissue formation and recovery.

Then we're going to have several more meals before we hit about 8 hours of food intake that must contain glycaemic index carbohydrates and proteins. If a person wishes to practice intermittent fasting during the seven days of the week and there are days when he does not exercise, the ideal for health purposes and to maintain insulin levels low is to reduce the amount of carbohydrate during the rest days and increase the amount of fat to have the elevated metabolic pathway of AMPK. It should be noted that fasting would not be one of the best strategies in high-performance athletes or people who eat very high calories throughout the day or are in the process of muscle hypertrophy, because in these situations you need to consume very high calories (especially carbohydrates) to have maximum glycogen levels and may cause problems at the intestinal level. Nevertheless, to boost hormonal levels and bowel functions, high-level athletes may benefit from one or two days a week of fasting.

Intermittent fasting is a technique of weight loss that involves interposing fasting periods with feeding periods. Not only "mere mortals" use this routine: athletes also use this form to remove fats that hinder their bodies.

Thanks to its simplicity, the diet is extremely popular. The approach is simply to disrupt food consumption over a certain period.

It forces the body to use its fat "reserves" to protect the biological unit. The body begins to lose weight slowly in this cycle of eating reserves.

It seems like a simple diet to do, but if you want to practice intermittent fasting, some specifics will make a difference.

Chapter Eleven

YOUR BODY CHANGES WITH INTERMITTENT FASTING

FROM 50 YEARS OLD

During the 50s, women begin to suffer from menopause, which is the absence of menstruation for more than 12 months and is due to the permanent cessation of follicular function. Its diagnosis is clinical and retrospective when 12 months have elapsed since the last period without any menstrual bleeding.

Lucas's conception clarifies that "there are no clear guidelines on how to deal with it because each woman has different experiences, but most of the changes in their bodies are related to it." During this period, the alteration in the distribution of body fat continues. The appearance of the skin in terms of elasticity and hydration worsens; vaginal dryness and other mucous membranes that can cause pain during sexual intercourse are experienced; muscle tone decreases, and muscle damage deteriorates. Bones of the spine, joints, or osteoarthritis problems appear.

"It also increases cardiovascular risk, sleep and memory disorders influenced by the gradual loss of estrogen," explains the specialist, adding that lifestyle changes can cause several mood changes: "during this stage, it is normal to suffer more anxiety, depression and a decrease in mood."

In the fifth decade, the woman may also notice that she loses pubic and axillary hair and undergoes changes in hair and skin or increases in body weight.

Menopause causes that; between 50 and 60 years, the woman's skin experiences many alterations. "The decrease in estrogen that occurs at this time in the woman's life leads to a thinning of the skin and dehydration, which causes wrinkles to intensify and 'sagging' of structures.

You should try acclimatizing the body to the symptoms of menopause by reducing body temperature with light clothing, drinking cold drinks and exercising regularly to prevent osteoporosis. Proper nutrition, doing controlled breathing exercises, going to gynecological exams, and other medical check-ups are also tipping to keep in mind during this stage and during the sixth decade of our life.

The specialist also recalls that throughout the woman's life, the gynecologist must be present, adapting her actions to the different health and reproductive status.

At every stage of the woman, physical changes and psychological changes occur, so that the specialist must be a foothold to ask constantly.

"These are vital phases that must be accepted and lived. You don't understand or doubt you have; you will have your gynecologist to solve them.

PROCESS OF THE CHANGE OF OUR BODY AND THE STATE OF WELL-BEING

Our health and well-being have taken priority in our daily lives: when we have free time, outside of work and when we are not occupied with occupations, we like to devote ourselves to activities that are healthy and fun: spending time with friends, playing sports, attending social gatherings, or participating in cultural activities, for example.

But, how do we go about attaining mental and physical well-being that will allow us to enjoy life every day and reach our full potential? We learn about new ways to promote our physical and mental health every day, but much information is still out there, and we may not have as much time as we deserve to familiarize ourselves with our health. Therefore, we are featuring a compilation of the best methods to help you feel physically and mentally healthy.

BREAK WITH A SEDENTARY LIFESTYLE

It does sound a bit cliché, but our way of life is exceptionally sedentary. At times we find ourselves suffering from the stagnation that could lead to depression because we are not taking advantage of our bodies and our surroundings (or, without going too far, to procrastinate and waste our free time, making us feel that we do not give up or take advantage of the time we have been given). Getting out into the world is an excellent way to escape this vicious cycle. This simple action could mean a considerable change in our mental state, especially for those who make it happen physically (something that always produces a feeling of health that raises our mood). Make sure you spend some time outside every day. If you spend this much time exercising in the fresh air each day, you should be able to smell the difference in your skin and hair in a few weeks. Walking is one of the healthiest exercises, and it burns the same calories as running, but it requires more effort because we walk faster. Relax and clear the mind.

TRY NEW CULTURAL ACTIVITIES

This may sound like an exaggeration, but every day of our lives we have the opportunity to experience new things. It is common for travelers to participate in cultural activities that enrich their travel experience. There are activities like watching plays, attending concerts and participating in cultural fairs where one can meet and learn about other cultures, explore different cultural movements of one's own country, and discover new ones.

PLAY SPORTS

To have a complete and healthy lifestyle, people must engage in regular exercise, maybe playing sports. There are ways to improve both mental and emotional well-being. However, getting physically fit not only occurs in training but is also a way to gain benefits in other areas of life.

—

Conducting exercise not only loosens our bodies but also exercises them, preventing them from atrophying. Another benefit of muscle growth is that it helps our physical appearance, and that, in turn, helps individuals to have a greater sense of self-confidence.

Beyond this, sport also offers a period of a shared company in the weekly routine that greatly benefits the individual. It offers opportunities for both work and play, enhancing social interaction in a very positive way. Regardless, physically fit people can practice physical exercise alone or in their home, doing various exercise routines every day. Keep in mind that physical exercise causes endorphins to be produced, which is the same as feeling happy while doing it.

New Experiences (EXTREME SPORTS)

You can also try out some new types of physical activities that can contribute to your workout routine while also discovering a new skill within yourself. An example is the aerial fabrics, which are in style now and can be practiced in a sports center or at home, and the wind tunnel, in which we can simulate what it is like to practice skydiving. We have in this line the type of sports where you take all of your adrenaline, and these are known as adrenaline sports. Also, you have sports like bungee jumping or any form of extreme sport that enables you to leave your stress behind and face something new.

Establish Routines

Routines are the groundwork for a healthy life and a satisfying existence. In reality, the volume of chaos we experience hourly does not lead to greater fullness in our life. Instead, it creates a fluctuating and disordered system in which our

---

daily schedule for hunger and sleep becomes thrown off. This can lead to insomnia (a very serious problem today). It may be that a system aids thinking systematically because it encourages the standardization of daily tasks and aids in creating an organized and well-structured manner of thinking focused on a particular objective. By creating schedules and routines, we can maximize the time that we have to complete our work. This helps us accomplish our duties faster and makes it easier to cope with our stress.

CULTIVATE HOBBIES AND HAVE HABITS

Our hobbies are a representation of our personality, which means exploring our hobbies is a way of learning more about ourselves. A fantastic way to commune with ourselves every day is to regularly explore new hobbies, as well as our current ones. Doing so will also help us forge new friendships, which are a key component to maintaining our overall well-being.

Stay Away From Bad Company and Consult Your Concerns with a Specialist

To cultivate emotional and mental health, the most important point is to understand ourselves. To stay mentally and physically fit, we must allow our brain to recuperate after periods of stress or take advantage of help when we require it. Considering our problems with a mental health professional (like a psychologist) is a great way to help maintain our overall mental and emotional well-being; it's like having a periodic physical health check-up. Alternatively, to take a step away from corporations that use up our resources and influence our daily lives for the worse, we must leave them behind to strengthen our positivity. Indeed, it is possible to improve your physical and mental health. The suggestions listed here can help you on your path to living a full life every-day.

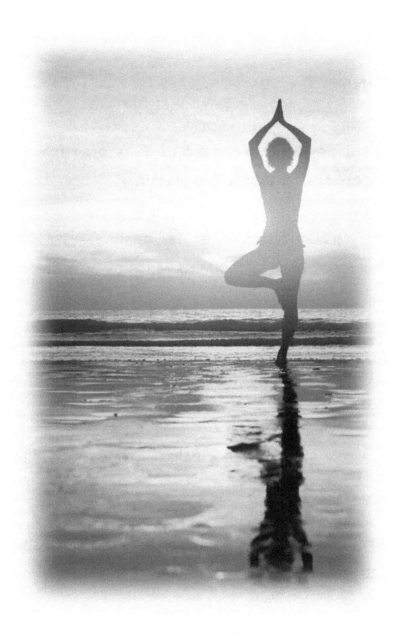

Chapter Twelve

What Foods to Avoid and Tips on How to Safely Do Intermittent Fasting

The chosen foods must be healthy, avoiding processed or fatty foods as much as possible:

- Candy;
- Industrialized cookies;
- Frozen or canned foods;
- Ready sauces;
- Whole dairy products;
- Refined cereals (including rice and white bread);
- Fried snacks;

Also, it is recommended not to use too much salt and sugar in the preparation of food.

FACILITATE YOUR NEW EATING PLAN

While it can be tempting to go directly into your new eating routine (the initial excitement is real), it can be difficult and make you hungrier and more uncomfortable. It is best to start slowly, doing two to three days of intermittent fasting during the first week, and then "gradually increasing week by week".

KNOW THE DIFFERENCE BETWEEN WHEN TO EAT AND WANTING TO EAT

After hearing your stomach growl, it may seem like there is no way to go more than X hours without food. Understand this question: ask yourself whether hunger is boredom or real hunger. If you are bored, get distracted by another task.

If you are really hungry but don't feel weak or dizzy (which are signs you should stop fasting as soon as possible), have a hot mint tea, as mint is known to reduce your appetite, or drink water with lemon (don't add sugar) to help fill your stomach until your next meal.

Now, if you have been trying to do intermittent fasting for some time and still feel extreme hunger between periods, you need to think about it. You need to add more nutrient-or calorie-rich foods over the eight hours or consider that this may not be the best plan for you. The addition of healthy fats, such as nuts, peanut, avocado, coconut butter, and olive oil, as well as protein, during the feeding period, can help keep you satisfied and full longer.

How to Do Intermittent Fasting: Eat When Needed

Technically, intense hunger and fatigue should not occur when following the 16: 8 fasting method (perhaps the most common). But if you feel extremely dizzy, you are probably low on sugar and need to eat something.

By definition, fasting involves removing some, if not all, food. Your best bet? Make a protein-rich snack, like a few slices of turkey breast or one to two hard-boiled eggs (to help you stay in a ketogenic (fat-burning) state. You can return to fasting, of course, if you want.

MOISTURIZE, HYDRATE, AND HYDRATE

Even when fasting, drinking water and drinks such as coffee and tea (without milk) are not only allowed, but especially in the case of H2O, encouraged. She recommends setting reminders throughout the day and, especially during fasting periods, to absorb lots of fluids. Try to fill at least 2, if not 3, liters per day.

BREAK YOUR FAST SLOWLY AND STEADILY

After several hours without food, you can feel like a human vacuum ready to suck what's on your plate. But killing the urge in minutes is not good for your body, according to research.

Instead, chew well and eat slowly to allow the digestive system to process food fully.

How to Do Intermittent Fasting: Avoid Overeating

Just because you have stopped fasting does not mean you should fill yourself with food. Eating cannot only make you bloated and uncomfortable, but it can also sabotage the weight loss goals that probably led you to intermittent fasting in the first place. Simply put: it's not necessarily how much of your plate can help you stay full longer, but what's on your plate.

Keep Balanced Meals

Having a healthy mix of proteins, fibers, healthy fats and carbohydrates can help you lose pounds and avoid extreme hunger when fasting. A good example? Grilled chicken with half a small sweet potato and sautéed spinach with garlic and olive oil.

When it comes to fruits, you want to opt for those with a low glycaemic index, which is digested, absorbed, and metabolized more slowly, causing a lower and slower increase in blood glucose. A stable blood sugar level helps prevent cravings-and therefore is critical when it comes to successfully losing weight.

PLAY WITH DIFFERENT PERIODS

Although Hertz mainly recommends 16:8, you need to look at your overall lifestyle to see which fasting method can best fit. For example, if you wake up early, it may be best to eat during the early hours, such as 10 am to 6 pm, and fast until the next morning at 10 am. Remember: The beauty of fasting is that it is easily changeable and flexible to your schedule.

Another option is to stop fasting early and have breakfast every day to increase your strength gradually. We all naturally fast once a day-while we sleep-so maybe you do 'close the kitchen' early. For example, "close" the kitchen at 9 pm and don't eat again until breakfast at 8 am. This is an 11-hour natural fast!

How to Do Intermittent Fasting: Avoid 24-Hour Fasting

Most nutritionists do not recommend fasting for an entire day, as this can lead to weakness, hunger, and increased food consumption-therefore weight gain.

If your goal is to lose weight, considering your total calorie intake and working to reduce that weight may be more beneficial than fasting for a long time (especially if you're the type who likes to eat afterward.)

Adapt Your Exercise Routine

You can exercise if you are on a fasting diet. But you have to be aware of what types of moves you make and when. If you choose to exercise on a fast, it is preferable to do it early in the morning, when you have more energy.

Nevertheless, while you are fasting, you are not feeding your muscles properly. So, you are more likely to get hurt. Consider lower impact exercises, such as yoga or steady-state cardio, on fasting mornings, and do HIIT class after eating.

KEEP CONTROL

Believe it or not, keeping a food diary can help you with your fasting diet. Actively write down details such as emotions and symptoms (level of hunger, weakness, etc.) that arise during intermittent fasting. This can help you assess your progress. You can also write down any trigger points that make fasting more difficult, such as drinking the night before.

LISTEN TO YOUR BODY

This is essential! Maintain awareness of dizziness, fatigue, irritability, headache, anxiety, and difficulty concentrating. When you have any of these situations, break your fast. This confirms that the body is in starvation mode and requires nourishment. And if you begin to feel cold, it is a sign to end the fast.

Additionally, be patient. While fasting, you may feel hungrier and weaker while fasting than usual. It is okay to have these feelings for up to a week. You should abandon the diet if these difficulties last longer and if you experience similar symptoms. Do not get sick!

Chapter Thirteen
Supplements and Intermittent Fasting

Intermittent fasting consists of alternating periods of feeding with others of fasting. Depending on the hours that we extend the time without eating, we will carry out one type of fast. The most common are 10 or 12 hours of fasting but it can also be extended to 24 hours.

According to different research, with 10 to 16 hours of fasting, the body already begins to notice the benefits of this resource, converting its fat reserves into energy and releasing ketones into the bloodstream.

It is important to include supplements that do not interfere with it or even help us make it more bearable during our fasting stage. These supplements can help us improve energy, reduce hunger and even give us a feeling of general well-being.

After getting to know the different intermittent fasting protocols and knowing how this diet can affect your body and mind, learn how to potentiate its effects through supplements. But first, an important warning: for your weight loss to be even more effective, do your workouts immediately before breaking your fast, so that right after the exercises you can eat. This strategy optimizes the recovery and synthesis of proteins and replenishes their energies.

Top Supplements for Intermittent Fasting
BCAA'S

When you are in a fasted state, you cannot have anything with calories. This can be very difficult when you are having a bad day and feeling hungry. It can also cause unnecessary muscle breakdown to support the body. Enter BCAAs— the savior of both problems. Branched Chain Amino Acids will have 0 calories and will prevent muscle breakdown when consumed. They will help fill you up so you can get to your food window.

BCAAs include leucine, and since it suppresses muscle breakdown, a BCAA supplement helps preserve muscle while you train in a fasted state.

Why not eat protein instead, you ask? Because food will increase your insulin levels and you will no longer be fasting. Whey protein is more insulinogenic than white bread.

BCAAs, on the other hand, have less of an impact on insulin levels than food, allowing you to fast while you train. That is why many people "in the know" supplement with them before fasting exercise.

FAT BURNER

Most people who use IF choose to do so to lose weight. Do you want to amplify this process and keep your body energized? Enter a fat burner. This will help keep your mood and energy levels up while supporting MORE fat loss.

Yohimbine HCL (please ask for doctor's approval before taking it) is a strong compound that can assist with fat loss while on a fasting schedule. It is a stimulant that helps increase adrenaline and dopamine levels in the body; and this can cause an increase in alertness and feelings of well-being.

Up to 0.2 mg/kg of body weight is recommended. That means a 150 lb person (divided by 2.2 to get kg) weighs 68kg and would work up to a dose of 14mg Yohimbine HCl or five capsules of Nutra BIO Yohimbine HCl a day.

Supplementation is most effective between meals or short-term fasting (empty stomach), you can divide the dose into 1 to 4 doses per day.

Example of other burners that you can use: Thermofield from Nutra BIO, is a complete fat burner since it also helps you control your hunger, increases energy, helps you with fatigue, and helps keep sugar levels stable. It's a simple formula, but as effective as Lipov 6 Black Ultra Concentrate.

MASS GAINERS (FOR BUILDING MUSCLE)

It becomes difficult to maintain a caloric surplus when you are on intermittent fasting. The window's purpose is to keep calories low and maximize nutrient absorption. To maximize your gains, you must consume enough calories. For a delicious, protein-rich mass gainer, look no further. Add it between meals and you will get an extra 300-900 calories for muscle-building. We suggest you take these supplements only if you do physical activity.

PRE-WORKOUT

If you DO and you exercise in the morning, you NEED some pre. You will need that kick in the gym since you are fasting. You just have to be careful and find a pre-workout that has 0 calories.

A suitable pre-workout fasting supplement will contain (at a minimum) caffeine and beta-alanine with minimal or no sugar. May also contain coralline, L-arginine, and creatine monohydrate.

These ingredients work together to increase muscular endurance, muscle power, focus, blood flow, and performance.

MULTI-VITAMIN

It is challenging to get three meals into your window to eat. Restricting caloric intake has a similar effect as restricting meals. Missing out on essential nutrients or vitamins for muscle building is possible. Intermittent fasting and daily multivitamins are mutually beneficial.

VITAMIN D

While prolonged fasting poses an increased risk of Vitamin D deficiency, it is still something intermittent fasting should pay attention to. Vitamin D is essential for immune health and it also helps the body absorb other essential nutrients like magnesium.

ELECTROLYTES

An important group of nutrients lost during long, intermittent fasts are electrolytes. When you are in a fasted state, ketone levels in your body increase, causing insulin levels to drop and essential nutrients are removed from the body. Although the numerous roles played by electrolytes, including sodium, magnesium, chloride, phosphate, potassium, calcium, and bicarbonate, are varied, they are essential for the nervous and muscular systems. A proper balance of electrolytes is also critical for ketogenesis, the process of converting fat into energy.

Depending on the type (s) of electrolytes missing, the symptoms of electrolyte deficiency can vary. These symptoms include:

- Nausea
- Fatigue
- Threw up
- Muscle weakness/spasms
- Headaches

- Irregular heartbeat

The possibility of low electrolyte symptoms causing a significant problem for those on a fast should be considered. An electrolyte imbalance and its symptoms can be avoided by ensuring you are giving your body enough of these essential nutrients while you are fasting.

Increasing the potassium, sodium, and magnesium levels are the most important electrolytes to supplement while on an intermittent fasting regimen. Without these three elements, which are easy to eliminate when fasting, our bodies would be deficient in the substances that maintain the proper balance of fluids and keep our blood pressure stable.

MAGNESIUM AND PROBIOTICS

Magnesium is a mineral found in various foods such as seeds, peanuts, and milk. It performs various functions in the body, such as regulating the functioning of nerves and muscles and helping to control blood sugar.

The daily recommendation for magnesium consumption is usually easily achieved when eating a balanced and varied diet, but in some cases, it may be necessary to use supplements, which must be prescribed by the doctor or nutritionist.

What is magnesium for?

Magnesium performs functions in the body such as:

Improves physical performance, because it is important for muscle contraction;

Prevents osteoporosis, because it helps to produce hormones that increase bone formation;

Helps to control diabetes, because it regulates the transport of sugar;

Decreases the risk of heart disease, as it decreases the accumulation of fatty plaques in blood vessels;

Relieves heartburn and poor digestion, especially when used in the form of magnesium hydroxide;

Controls blood pressure, especially in pregnant women at risk for eclampsia.

In addition, magnesium is also used in laxative medications to fight constipation and in medications that act as antacids for the stomach.

Magnesium-rich foods

Foods rich in magnesium are usually also high in fiber, with the main ones being whole grains, legumes, and vegetables. See the full list:

Legumes, such as beans and lentils;

Whole grains, such as oats, whole wheat, and brown rice;

Fruits, such as avocado, banana, and kiwi;

Vegetables, especially broccoli, pumpkin, and green leaves, such as kale and spinach;

Seeds, especially the pumpkin and sunflower seeds;

Oilseeds, such as almonds, hazelnuts, Brazil nuts, cashew nuts, peanuts;
Milk, yogurt, and other derivatives;
Others: coffee, meat, and chocolate.

Magnesium Supplements

Magnesium supplements are usually recommended in cases of deficiency of this mineral, being possible to use both a multivitamin supplement in general containing magnesium and the magnesium supplement, which is normally used in the form of chelated magnesium, magnesium aspartate, magnesium citrate, magnesium lactate, or magnesium chloride.

Supplementation should be indicated by the doctor or nutritionist, as the recommended dose depends on the factor causing your deficiency, in addition, its excess can cause nausea, vomiting, hypotension, drowsiness, double vision, and weakness.

PROBIOTICS

Probiotics are foods or supplements that contain live microorganisms intended to maintain or enhance the "good" bacteria (normal microbiota) in the body. Prebiotics are foods (generally high in fiber) that act as nutrients for the human microbiota and are used with the intention of improving the balance of these microorganisms.

Probiotics are found in foods like yogurt, sauerkraut, whole grains, bananas, green leafy vegetables, onions, garlic, soybeans, and artichokes. Additionally, probiotics and prebiotics are added to some foods and are available as dietary supplements.

The gut microbiota's connection to disease is being researched. The health benefits of probiotics and prebiotics currently available have not been proven conclusively.

However, side effects are uncommon, and most healthy adults can safely consume prebiotics and probiotics-containing foods. Future research could lead to more advanced probiotics with greater health benefits.

Essential Nutrients after 50 Years

To get the most out of your 50s, you have to keep increasing your nutrient intake as you age. Once a person's body has finished going through certain changes, a series of important events occur in their bodily system, which influences many vital organs' functioning. It is critical to follow a healthy diet to help prevent the development of chronic illnesses.

Whether or not you already know this, I think you should be aware that dietary requirements change with age and lifestyle. Athletes, for example, require a higher level of carbohydrates than people who are not involved in regular physical activity. Just as is the case with nutritional needs in general, the amount of nutrients required through diet differs depending on the individual's age.

Once you have discovered the nutrients you should be concerned about, you will find out which of those nutrients are crucial in your diet because of their health effects. But if you do have any questions, please consult your trusted nutritionist.

CALCIUM

A calcium deficiency can lead to bone problems. It has been shown to help prevent bone fractures, which is why you should keep ingesting them.

However, this nutrient is much more important in women than in men. This is because, after menopause, they are more likely to develop osteoporosis due to hormonal changes.
On the other hand, it is necessary to ensure that vitamin D levels are adequate. This substance plays a key role in allowing calcium to be absorbed at the intestinal level, where it then

makes its way to the bone tissue and then it must carry out its essential functions.

B12 Vitamin

Vitamin B12 is essential in the differentiation of red blood cell lines. Anemia occurs without this compound, causing extreme fatigue and tiredness. According to a study in the Medical Clinics of North America, "megaloblastic anemia" was once known as "metaphosphate osteodystrophy".

Developing a disease like this could have a significant impact on lifestyle habits. To ensure that the requirements are met, simply include animal-based foods in the diet regularly.

Protein

It has been commonly claimed that high-protein diets are bad for the liver and kidneys. However, current evidence disputes this.

Some nutrients must be increased in the diet by the age of 50 to preserve lean mass, as suggested by research. A daily protein intake of 1.4 grams per kilogram of bodyweight might be ideal.

Remember that the ingested proteins must be 50% of high biological value. All essential amino acids and a good digestibility value must be present. Also, those who are from animal-based foods exhibit both characteristics.

Foods That You Should Consider In Your Diet after 50 Years

It is necessary to highlight certain foods in the diet to avoid deficiencies that may negatively affect health.

MEAT AND FISH

The taste for meat and fish does diminish after age, and the preference for these meats wanes as one gets older, but it is imperative to keep up a consistent diet of meat and fish to maintain proper nutrition. These products contain high-quality proteins and essential micronutrients, like iron, that can avoid the risk of anemia.

Eggs

Eggs were once believed to increase cholesterol and raise LDL (bad cholesterol) levels, but now the myth has been debunked. Even if these foods may not influence the body's lipid profile or the risk of cardiovascular disease, they don't appear to increase cardiovascular disease risk.

Also, they supply amino acids and fats which help with promoting a healthy state of well-being. Finally, they have vitamin D, a nutrient that is severely lacking in a large segment of the population. It is recommended to consume at least 5 servings of it each week.

GREEN LEAFY VEGETABLES

Green Leafy vegetables are known to contain phytonutrients and vitamin C in their composition. While each element is required for proper bodily functions, it is equally important to ensure proper bodily reactions each day.

It should be noted that this vitamin is an essential nutrient that keeps the immune system in an operational state and thus keeps different infectious diseases at bay.

Tips and Aspects to Consider for a Good Diet after 50 Years

You can still include foods as you age; however, other health strategies should be considered, such as increasing the frequency of consumption or choosing specific foods to increase intake.

PRACTICE INTERMITTENT FASTING

Fasting has been proven to improve insulin resistance and reduce fat levels in those who follow it. Most people can benefit from them, though they are not ideal for everyone. To be sure, consulting with a professional is always a good idea.

MELATONIN SUPPLEMENTS

Melatonin is a neurohormone synthesized in the pineal gland and regulating sleep-wake cycles. From the age of 50, its production drops dramatically, which can condition the quality of rest.

To avoid having the condition, you should ingest it externally. Consumption of 1.8 milligrams of the substance 30 minutes before going to sleep helps reduce the number of interruptions that happen during the night. Additionally, it is a powerful antioxidant, which has beneficial effects on the promotion of pathologies comprised of several factors.

CONSUME FERMENTED FOODS

The intestinal microbiota undergoes a variety of changes as the years go by. The change in the diversity of species that occurs over time may alter digestive function.

Thus, it is essential to consume fermented dairy, such as yogurt or kefir regularly. The good bacteria found in these foods are capable of colonizing different areas of the digestive tract. As a result, they can benefit the host's overall health.

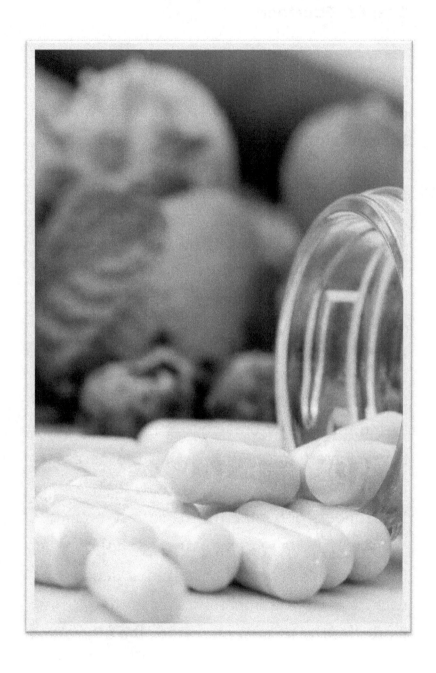

Chapter Fourteen

Good habits during the intermittent fasting and things you can co to get back to Your Ideal Weight

Breakfast

The first meal of the day has to be used to replenish all the energy used during the hours of sleep. Also, it also prepares the body for the day of physical and mental effort that is about to start.

Specialists recommend not skipping any meal and in the case of breakfast, it is essential. You have to start the day by taking the necessary nutrients.

It is understood that the healthiest breakfast consists of dairy food, fruit, and cereals. However, this is not a closed rule, it depends on each person. The important fact is that it must be as healthy as possible. As for the schedules, you should have breakfast as early as possible. It is best not to do it after 10.

Lunch at Noon

Some specialists maintain that the best time to eat the "third" (not the "second") meal of the day is between 1:00 and 3:00 p.m.

Eating high-calorie meals after 3 p.m. can be particularly counterproductive. This is because the process of digesting food becomes more inefficient so you could gain more weight. The latest research suggests that eating too early may reduce the risk of gaining fat mass.

At Night You Have to Prepare to Sleep

Just as breakfast should be forceful to gather energy for the day to begin, dinner should be the lightest of all meals of the day.

It is healthier to have an early dinner to give your body time to digest. Also, fish or lean meats are recommended, accompanied by some dairy (as long as we do not have gastric problems.)

Food intakes after 10 pm can make us gain a little more weight and, also, cause nightmares and insomnia problems.

About Desserts, Fruits, Coffee, and Snacks

Desserts are usually always in the spotlight when talking about diets, losing weight, or not gaining weight.

Some assure that they should be banished from the menu without any contemplation.

There are fewer radical opinions, which argue that they can be eaten in moderation, however, in no case, after any of the three main meals.

In the case of desserts, it is recommended to take them first thing in the morning, since before noon the body processes carbohydrates much better.

Another good time is just before starting any physical activity. Thus, you will fill the body with energy, without forcing the stomach too much.

One tip becoming fashionable is to have a piece of fruit before eating and not as a dessert. This can be a good way to decrease hunger and feeling, besides, to achieve a satiating effect.

Good Hydration: as Important as Eating

There is no healthy diet if you don't consume enough water. This helps us feel more satiated, which can help us lose weight. Besides, it also contributes in a certain way to the metabolism of fats.

Specialists also recommend certain times for this:

- Two glasses of water as soon as you wake up to cleanse the body.
- A glass half an hour before the main meals, as well as before bathing and sleeping.

In total, you should consume between a litter and a half and two liters of water a day. However, these schedules alone do not work. We must combine them with a balanced diet and regular exercise.

Avoid Consuming Sugar

It is generally known that sugary foods are a significant contributor to obesity. Conversely, since they increase the risk of diabetes, obesity, and heart disease, they also cause them.

Tips

- Replace refined sugar with healthy sweeteners like honey or stevia.
- Read the labels of the foods you buy at the grocery store and make sure they are low in sugar and saturated fat.
- Calm your sweet tooth with "light" desserts or nuts.

EAT A GOOD BREAKFAST

Not eating a good breakfast everyday makes it difficult to regain your ideal weight. Not only have those who avoid the food run the risk of being overweight, but their physical and mental well-being also suffer.

Tips

- Make sure you prepare a complete and balanced breakfast, which corresponds to 25% of your total daily calories.
- Eat plenty of fruits, vegetables, and complex carbohydrate sources.
- Don't forget a small helping of healthy fats and protein.

INCREASE YOUR WATER INTAKE

Water helps to improve your figure and body weight in many ways. Since much of the body is made up of this fluid, it is essential for metabolism and an optimal detoxification process.

Tips

- Drink between 3 and 4 liters of water a day.
- If you do not want to drink only water, supplement your fluid intake with herbal teas, natural juices, or fruits rich in water.
- On hot days or when doing sports activities, increase your consumption.

Get a Good Night's Sleep to Return to Your Ideal Weight

To successfully lose weight, ensure you do not skip any rest days. Despite appearing to be unrelated, sleep plays a central role in metabolic functions and all weight-loss-related processes.

Tips

- Try to sleep without interruptions for 7 or 8 hours a day.
- Avoid distractions before sleeping so as not to shorten the rest period.
- Have a light dinner so that you do not have digestive discomfort when going to bed.

Avoid Zero Carbohydrate Diets

Reducing carbohydrate consumption has interesting effects in controlling overweight. However, it is not advisable to eliminate them from the diet. These macronutrients are a major source of energy that should be incorporated into any meal plan.

Tips

- Instead of choosing simple carbohydrates (bread, pastries, flours, etc.) opt for complex carbohydrate sources (oatmeal, brown rice, quinoa, etc.)

- Try to consume them only for breakfast and lunch.

Divide the Portions of Food

Large plates are not a good option for a healthy and slimming diet. While they are satisfying for the moment, they overload digestion and slow metabolism. The best option is to divide the servings by five or six meals a day.

Tips

- Eat small meals every 3-4 hours.
- Choose to have 3 main meals and 2 snacks.

REDUCE THE SALT

To return to your ideal weight, you must avoid salt. Although this condiment is commonly used in the kitchen, overconsumption affects negatively both health and figure. Too much salt causes high blood pressure, inflammation, and fluid retention.

Tips

- Use herbs and spices to enhance the flavor.
- Do not use your favorite products if they contain a lot of sodium.

Get Physical Exercise

Regular physical exercise is the best complement to your diet. This type of activity starts the metabolism and optimizes the energy burn. Therefore, following a training routine or playing sports is very beneficial.

How to Use Intermittent Fasting Benefits to Better Your Life

Scientists have found many advantages of intermittent fasting to reduce caloric intake for one cause or another. With this approach, the body will adjust several characteristics for the better. The real question is not if fasting can help you or not, but how it will help you and how often you should.

This fasting style has been shown to lower blood pressure and increase levels of HDL. It can help greatly with diabetes management and will also help you lose weight. All these effects sound pretty good and can be achieved with the fasting of this type. Studies carried out on several different animal species show that limiting caloric intake increases their lives by 30 percent. Human studies show it reduces blood pressure, blood sugar, and sensitivity to insulin. With these experiments, fasting would improve a human's life if performed for an extended period. Cutting the calories by 30 percent all the time will achieve the same results, but this has been shown to cause depression and irritability. Fasting is a method offered instead of simply cutting calories and it has benefits without stress or irritability.

Intermittent fasting works out every other day by eating food. You will end up eating nearly twice as much food on the days you eat as you normally would. You still get the same number of calories but you are also getting all the benefits. It will lower the levels of stress and improve your overall health. This kind of fasting is a great way of getting into better physical condition, living a longer life, and feeling better all the time.

DIET TO REDUCE STRESS AND INCREASE HAPPINESS

Stress and our body share a strong relationship For example, muscle tension is a reflex reaction to stress; it is the body's way of protecting itself against danger. It may feel like a little ache or something tightening in the back of your neck or lower back as you type on the computer. Headaches are a close cousin. The relationship is so strong that it has its term: stress headaches (also known as "tension pains.")

Stress even causes digestive problems as it alters the concentration of acid in the stomach that can lead to inflammation, colic, diarrhea, constipation, irritable bowel syndrome, and even peptic ulcers. Stress disrupts the body's insulin production, which can lead to diabetes and even heart attacks or strokes. Healthy diets have been shown to prevent these damaging physical effects of stress and even reverse the ageing process. Life is short, and your diet is an easy way to take control and maximize your well-being.

Eating a healthy diet will make you a more effective leader. You owe it to yourself to properly feed your body and brain, so here are four steps to creating a successful eating plan.

GIVE PRIORITY TO BREAKFAST

Starting the day well is important. You should get into the habit of eating breakfast. Skipping breakfast can make it difficult to maintain stable blood sugar levels. What you give to your body is also important. Try to choose foods high in fiber like cereals, oatmeal, whole wheat bread, and fresh fruit. High-fiber foods digest more slowly and keep you satisfied, as well as jump-start your metabolism and stabilize your blood sugar levels, allowing you to focus and reduce your anxiety and stress.

As a leader, breakfast may be the most important meal of the day, but it doesn't end there. Intermittent fasting for sugar control and weight loss can harm your mind and the relationships you have with your team. When you value the connection between your stomach and your mind, you get the most out of your day. The gift of life is quite short and fleeting.

Limit the Consumption of Refined Sugars and Processed Foods

Certain foods can harm your brain. Do not go near refined sugar. White sugar and high fructose corn syrup should be avoided. You should not give your team these foods, as you want them to be successful too.

Low-sugar diets have been shown to increase brain neurotrophic factor (BDNF), a peptide responsible for creating new neurons. This peptide makes neurons connect and combine, in addition to playing a fundamental role in neuroplasticity.

Try to avoid filling your kitchen with products high in sugar and foods with a high glycemic index such as bread, sweet drinks, and fast food. Better try fruit, honey, or maple syrup. Or better yet, go for a natural protein like soy that will help you build muscle. Refined sugars will give you a quick energy boost, but you'll soon feel like your blood sugar is on a roller coaster ride, not a fun one.

When sugar levels drop, your adrenal glands release stress hormones like cortisol. This will affect your performance as a leader. You will be more irritable in conversations; your relationships will suffer and you will not make the correct decisions that your team needs.

INCLUDE OMEGA-3 FATTY ACIDS

Omega-3 fatty acids are gifts for any leader and you deserve to include them in your diet. Nuts and seeds, including chia, flaxseed, and walnuts, are your best friends and partners. Nuts are known to protect the heart and contain antioxidants. Walnuts are particularly healthy and a rich source of omega-3 fatty acids that reduce the risk of heart attacks and bad cholesterol.

Omega-3 helps stabilize adrenal hormones and prevent them from spiking, especially when you're stressed, thus becoming a powerful antidote to stress.

LIMIT YOUR INTAKE OF CAFFEINE AND ALCOHOL

Craving caffeinated foods is natural. We all crave coffee, tea, soda, or chocolate, but it's important to recognize that these foods can affect our overall well-being. Caffeine stimulates the production of cortisol, the stress hormone. Having an occasional cup of coffee is fine, but try to avoid it before bed because it can give you insomnia. You should also think about when and how to consume alcohol. Alcohol is a depressant and sedative that alters neurotransmitters in the brain. Having a couple of beers or a couple of glasses of wine after work may sound tempting, but try not to overdo this habit because it could negatively affect your performance as a leader.

When you are stressed, it is easier to indulge in cravings and give in to impulses, facilitating drug or alcohol use as a defense mechanism. In the long term, this can result in addiction. It is best to avoid these temptations when you are experiencing high levels of stress.

Your eating habits and the level of stress you handle go hand in hand. When you're stressed, it's natural to crave comfort foods like desserts, fast food, and alcohol, but these foods can be addictive and wind you down a dead-end spiral. Fuelling your body for success will reduce stress, improve your productivity, and strengthen your relationship with your team, so keep these four steps in mind to create a high-performance eating plan.

TIPS TO START A HEALTHY LIFE

- Learn something new every day. Healthy entrepreneurs are eternal dreamers: They work hard, play hard and think hard. They love to read, listen to audiobooks, and absorb as much knowledge as possible. They educate themselves on topics relevant to their business and also seek knowledge of other types. They know that healthy behaviors have a direct impact on their business.

- Set goals and create systems to achieve them: Healthy entrepreneurs also understand that knowledge without application is the fastest path to failure. They go beyond learning-they apply. They realize that daily journeys and steps are the only way to achieve goals.

- If you want to make the most of your free time, spend it wisely: It is estimated the average person spends three hours per day watching television. That is a very kind thing of you to do, but please do not be that kind of person. To stay healthy, you should concentrate on growing your business, taking care of yourself and your family, and making the world a better place. Another piece of advice is to spend time or engage in meditation to gain a better sense of your goals.

- Make exercise a priority. A healthy body helps cultivate a healthy mind: An adult should exercise 2.5 hours a week or more with moderate to intense aerobic activity and two intensive training sessions a week. Even if you are very busy, find 10 minutes here and there. Doing so will help you relieve stress and get endorphins to overcome your business challenges.

- Eat less junk food. Think of food as fuel: The higher the quality of fuel you put in your tank, the better you will perform. You don't need to go on a diet to eat healthily. Only eat more real foods (that come from nature), instead of processed and fast food. Doing so will improve your energy level and mood, among other benefits.

- Get more sleep. All entrepreneurs experience sleepless nights, morning meetings, and last-minute deliveries. But a healthy entrepreneur knows that sleep is essential to their success. Whether you're getting up early and getting big projects done in the morning or you're hopelessly awake, find a consistent sleep routine and stick with it. Don't underestimate the power of a good nap to recharge your brain, either.

- Create a balance in your life: Healthy entrepreneurs treat their health as a lifestyle. You can't put a Band-Aid on a bad Business Plan, just like you can't eat healthy for a week and hope to lose weight. Successful entrepreneurs adopt a healthy lifestyle: They work smart, they don't work anymore.

Conclusion : How Intermittent Fasting Has Changed Me?

My intermittent fasting experience is very good; otherwise, I would not have kept it (and still do) for so long. Personally, it has given me very good results both in body composition and improving my relationship with food. Of course, those results come over time, when it's part of your lifestyle-they aren't overnight changes.

If we talk about body composition, intermittent fasting added to training (especially strength training,) and a healthy diet, it has allowed me to maintain a good muscle mass level and reduce my percentage of body fat. In the times when I have strictly followed training and nutrition, I have managed to go down to approximately 16.5%; But, more importantly, in times when I have to reduce workouts for any issue, I have stayed without problems at around 20% without much effort and maintaining a good base of lean mass.

Regarding the relationship with food, intermittent fasting has helped me to notably reduce my anxiety when it comes to eating: knowing that I have established times to eat and that, within them, I eat when I'm hungry (without having to " wait for lunch or dinner ") has also made that anxiety to relax and learn to differentiate the" physical hunger "of the" emotional hunger ". I do not have the feeling at any time of "being on a diet", but of having some routines and sticking to them as part of my day today.

It is important to note two facts that have also been helpful to me whenever I have practiced intermittent fasting: on the one hand, the fact of being flexible, especially during weekends, when sometimes I do not comply with the same schedules as the days of diary. As I said above, it is important that the diet or, in this case, the nutritional strategy, adapts to us, and not us to it.

On the other hand, we have a healthy diet most of the time with specific whims. Intermittent fasting is of little use, especially if we seek to improve our health through it if we base our diet on ultra-processed and other unhealthy products. Maintaining a healthy diet is essential if we want to achieve the benefits that this alternative promises us.

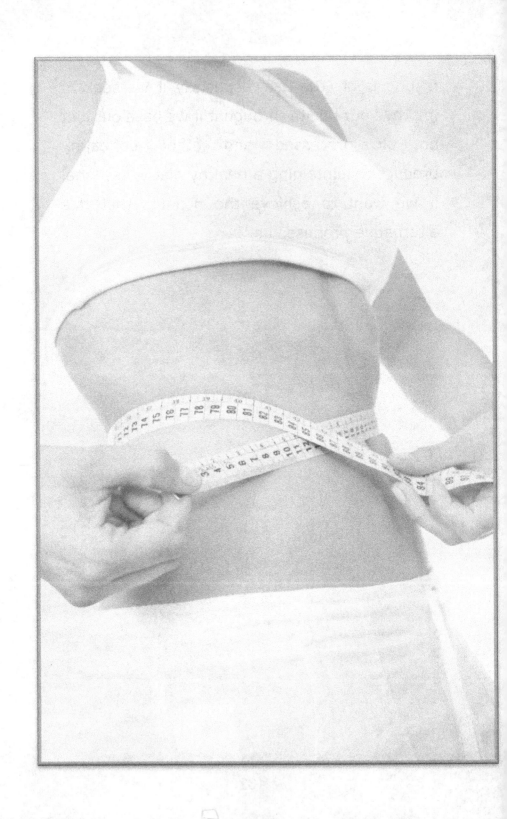